Common

Sense

For

Good

Health

&

Longevity

Also by Andrew S.S. Chan

The Invisible Rings
At the Tea House
Are We Lucky or What

To our children: Marcie and Garwin

Also to: All the folks who are kind and generous enough to share their health secrets with me for this book.

Introduction

This book is about my personal journey to good health. It is not meant to be medical advice given by a health professional. But, all the common senses mentioned here in this book could be useful to help you adopt a healthier daily routine in pursuit of good health and longevity.

Table of Contents

1

Why I Write this Book

This book is an accident. It evolved from a letter, intended for my two children a year or so ago, about how to stay healthy, physically, and mentally. Because they both have very demanding jobs and live in Hong Kong, one of the most dynamic parts of the world, my wife and I naturally worry about their health. Stressful jobs, unhealthy lifestyles, insufficient rest, and lack of exercise and relaxation might ruin their health permanently and shorten their lives. But, as I was writing the letter, I realized it would be too long of a letter if I were going to include all the things that I wanted them to know. In fact, it would be long enough to call it a book – a short one, at least. And, if I limit it to just a letter by leaving out some of the pertinent reasonings and facts, just telling them to "do this and do that or don't do this and don't do that" like a nagging mother, I'm sure they won't pay much attention to it. They're both intelligent adults now, and they won't easily accept any new or old ideas unless they are compellingly convincing.

Well, if the book is good enough for my children, then it should be good enough for other people too. And if I, through my book, can in any way help other people attain good health and longevity and live a happier life, then why not? It would be a good thing to do.

My Qualifications

A friend asked what qualifications I have to write this kind of book, thinking that I ought to be a medical doctor, a research professor, or at least a nutritionist in order to give advice on the subject. He, like many people, is a perfect follower – he doesn't think nor question and he underestimates his own intelligence and believes blindly in people with fame, authority, and a fancy title. It doesn't dawn on him that in this television and internet age, there are very few trustworthy sources that provide accurate and truthful information. Anyone with a computer or a smartphone can supply false information and post it on websites or social media. Anyone can proclaim an expert of this and that if he can afford to buy TV times to promote his program. For financial gains, so many offenders are willing to lie, cheat and even falsify credentials. Had my friend used his brain just a little bit more, he'd have checked out the sources and their providers, and then, he'd have known the truths: *facts speak louder than eloquent orations.*

First, let me clarify, this book is not a research report nor is it a thesis or a medical guidebook. It's all about *common sense – common* sense that has a lot to do with good health and longevity, and common sense that I've acquired from personal experiences of going through a serious illness and its ensuing long and painful recovery periods, of nurturing myself back to good health and, most importantly, of observing and talking to hundreds of healthy people who live a long and happy life. Surprisingly, quite a few of them were very sick when they were young and, like me, were able to reverse their luck simply by exercising good common sense. One friend is Mr. Small, even though he was much older than I. He and I were good friends for more than twenty years until he passed away three years ago at 96. Although his illness (a debilitating and painful nerve disorder) was not exactly like mine, his route to good health was almost the same, except his was many times more painful and difficult. His determination and courage not only enabled him to overcome his poor health, but also made him a very successful real estate investor. I owe much of my modest success to him, for his success story had inspired me.

I hope our experiences may also benefit you. But, if you already have good health, then you don't need to waste your time reading this book because you must have done all the right things for yourself. Otherwise, you won't be healthy. Your way may not be the same as ours, but it doesn't matter, as long as it works for you. That's the purpose of this book: to help those who are now unhealthy, just like I was, to find their own way back to a healthy and happy life.

Besides, many great books, music, fine arts, inventions, and philosophy are created by *common* people

3

like you and me and not by academics or professionals whose thinking are confined by the boundaries of their own narrow fields and are too arrogant to explore other alternatives. Furthermore, there are already plenty of books and TV programs on this popular subject of good health and longevity. Who doesn't want to have excellent health and live a long life? People, rich and poor, from ordinary citizens to kings and queens, have been chasing this elusive dream for thousands of years and no one has yet found the answer that fits us all. Even in this techno-logical age, with huge databases, lightning-fast comput-ers, and numerous researches on every conceivable sub-ject, including the study of many centenarians of the world, many are still hoping to find a consistent and relia-ble secret formula. Still, we haven't come up with any proven formula for good health and longevity other than making some minor improvements.

The reason for this is clear. Like our faces, we're all different – different in look, in genes, in digestive and immune systems, and even in the way we think. In addi-tion, we don't breathe the same air, eat the same food, and have the same families and friends sharing our daily lives. So, how can we, living in America, emulate to live as long and healthy as a few centenarians who spend all their lives living in the tiny fishing villages of Okinawa, Japan? Even if exact emulation is possible by relocating our-selves to Okinawa and living exactly the same way as those centenarians live, we still may not turn out to be centenarians ourselves because our genes are different. We may be healthier and possibly add a few more years to our lives due to better air quality and healthier lifestyle. Not all the residents in Okinawa are centenarians either; some of them die young, too. That demonstrates that diet and lifestyle are important for good health and longevity, but there are many other factors as well. In general, we live longer and have better health now than ever before, mainly because we have better nutrition, better healthcare, and more advanced medical technology. But, the gain is somewhat offset by polluted air and water, poisonous foods, and stresses that come with the fast-paced modern lifestyle.

Unfortunately, almost all the health and longevity books and programs ignore the reality of the conditions in modern life; they're based on theories, and their premises are rooted in perfect conditions, such as clean air and pure water, foods without chemicals, and stress-free environments. But, it's impossible to have these kinds of conditions unless we live a hermit life in a place far away from civilization. Our air is smoggy and our water and foods are loaded with poisonous chemicals, which are the primary causes of the various deadly diseases we have today. Thus, the health gurus' teachings are impractical and, therefore, impossible to follow. What makes things worse is that a good percentage of today's books and TV programs are not authored by experts. They're manufactured by opportunists who want to profit from the multi-billion dollars a year health industry geared towards the health-conscious consumers, who are hungry for advice and products which, in general, are not only useless, but also downright harmful.

This book, unlike other typical health books which provide a bundle of seemingly expert advice on everything imaginable, teaches you only *one* thing – to use *common sense*. Common sense can be developed by exercising your brain more often and can help you distinguish advice that makes sense from those that make no sense at all. The advantage of this "common sense" approach is that you can improve your health without spending extra money on equipment and dietary supplements, and without making radical changes in the way you're living now unless your current diet and lifestyle are extremely unhealthy. You don't need to quit your job and relocate to Okinawa and eat fish and vegetables only. You don't need to live like the Okinawans – three or four generations under the same roof. And, you don't need to grow your own vegetables and raise your own chickens. However, you still need the discipline and dedication to follow the rules of *moderation* and *consistency* and, most important of all, the *willpower* to resist the temptations of an unhealthy lifestyle. In short, you're your own boss, and you're the one who decides your own destiny.

2

My Experience

It is not my intention to bore you with my personal health problems, but I think it is important for you to understand that the good health I enjoy today is the direct result of the bad health I had when I was a youngster. The lessons I have learned by trial and error during that dark period of my life were invaluable and, I believe, my unfortunate experiences could be helpful should you encounter similar situations.

In 1961, when I was seventeen, I suddenly came down with a rare form of osteoarthritis, causing excruciating pain in my right hip. No doctors knew how and why I got it, but I had a feeling that it came from years of bodily abuses and sufferings during the period from 1949 to 1955 when I was living in China under the Communist regime. Like most people during that time, I was undernourished due to my family not having enough to eat. All we had on the table most of the time were cabbages, yams, pumpkins, potatoes, and rice. Even those were not enough to fill our empty stomachs. Meats were rare; we might have a little bit of pork once or twice a month. The only time we had beef was when a water buffalo was accidentally killed by lightning.

I was forced to attend a school far away from home to avoid bullying by other local boys because of my family background – we were labeled as "enemies of the people" just because my father had held an office with previous regime. At first, I lived in a relative's home, and later, I moved out (for reasons too personal and tedious to mention here) to live with four other boys in similar situations. We slept on desks put together at night as makeshift beds and put them back in the morning before classes started. Without any family or guardian supervision, we were living like wild animals; we regularly went to sleep hungry and in cold, damp clothes. And we, somehow, always got into fights with the local boys and had many bodily injuries which, except the more serious ones, were largely ignored due to our ignorance and childish toughness.

By 1964, nine years after my escape to Macau by swimming, my bad hip got so painful that I could hardly walk, and eventually, I had to quit school. My father, who loved me very much and was desperate to find a cure for me, spent a small fortune on my medical expenses, and I spent a lot of time at the doctors' offices. He indiscriminately listened to friends and relatives' recommendations and had me try out Western doctors, Chinese herbal doctors, acupuncturists, chiropractors, and even religious healers and ghost hunters. I visited the acupuncturist almost every day to let him probe around in the vicinity of my bad hip with a skinny long needle, searching for God-knows-what. I had hormone and cortisone shots once a week and I drank Chinese herbal medicines like soda pops and swallowed a myriad of painkillers like popcorn whenever the pain became unbearable. In addition to vitamins and other nutritious foods, I had all sorts of expensive and exotic foods added to my regular diet – ginseng tea, deer antler, tiger bone, bird's nest, shark fin, aged turtle, old hen, fish oil, poisonous snake gallbladder, and many more ridiculous things, of which my father honestly believed would help relieve my pain. The amount of medicine and health foods I consumed was enough to open a small pharmacy and a health food store. But all these efforts and money didn't do me any good, and my condition worsened. And, it was the many months of cortisone shots that weakened my immune system so much – to the point that a common cold I caught turned into pneumonia and put me in a hospital for many painful days, nearly killing me.

My first hospital experience served me well though; it woke me up and got me thinking, "Something is very wrong if all these exotic foods and medicines have not improved my health, but instead, have ruined it. I kept reminding myself, "I must quit them and find a better way to nurture myself back to good health." Common sense told me that I should quit thinking about my sickness, ignore the pains, and stop feeling sorry for myself that I was limping and couldn't go back to school. (My high school wouldn't hold the place for me for more than one year.)

With my father's unconditional love and support, I moved to our country house and bought a ten-speed bicycle. Every day, I rode leisurely on country roads to different places – usually to quiet and beautiful places – and spent time there drawing pictures or reading books. Miraculously, just by moving to the countryside, away from the city, away from the doctors and medicines, away from the acupuncturists and needles, and away from the old hens and snake gall bladders, and just by exposing myself to Mother Nature, soaking in the warm sun and breathing the fresh air, I was already feeling a lot better. Less than a year of country living, I became a healthy person again despite having a still bothersome bad hip. I found out years later in America that there was absolutely nothing I could do about it except to have hip replacement surgery. My right hip had been damaged beyond repair.

3

Healthy Traits and Habits

Maybe it is because I wasn't healthy when I was young; I have always admired people with good health and taken an interest in finding out their secrets. From very early on, I started talking to healthy old folks from different ethnic groups, social, and economic back-grounds. I have asked no less than a hundred of them over the years many questions regarding the food they eat, the places they live, their habits, daily routines, and lifestyles. By comparing and cross-referencing their answers, I have discovered that they have more than a few things in common: they all have a lot of common sense. They eat *moderately*, drink *sensibly*, exercise *selectively*, and they are *fun-loving* and *optimistic*. Most important of all, they are not choosy eaters and they keep themselves busy and are pleased with themselves.

Attaining good health is a form of competition for older people. When we were kids, we competed to be the one who had the newest toys. As teenage boys, we competed in owning the fastest bicycle, and for teenage girls, the prettiest dress. As young adults, we competed in what universities we attended and how good-looking our girl-friends or boyfriends were. When we became parents and entered middle age, we competed in what kind of car we drove and what kind of house we lived in. Later, we competed in how successful our children were. Now that we're old and all those things that we competed in are in the past and don't matter anymore, the only thing that matters now is our health. So, we compete in health, to see who is the healthiest. Health, which we have been taking for granted all our lives, has suddenly become the center of the competition, and good health has become the ultimate goal, the precious prize, and the measurement of a lifetime achievement that we can be proud of.

4

Definition of Good Health

Before I proceed to discuss how to attain good health and longevity, I must first define what "good health" is. Many people mix up good health with physical fitness, thinking that they are the same thing. They automatically consider you healthy if you are well-built – broad shoulders, thick chest, flat belly, muscular biceps, and thighs. They don't know, unless you've told them, that you have heart disease, diabetes, or a degenerated disc. They don't know that you must take painkillers to ease your back pains and sleeping pills to go to sleep. They don't know you are not healthy at all. It is not necessarily true that a big and muscular person who can lift two hundred pounds is healthier than a skinny one who has difficulty with twenty pounds. It couldn't be more wrong to assess a person's health condition simply by his appearance alone. Contrary to the general belief, an overly muscular person is more likely to be an unhealthy person – he is prone to heart diseases according to studies (there are many and their validities are debatable) because one can train and build other muscles easily, but not cardiac muscles. It is so tender that it just can't withstand the heavy strain of lifting 200 pounds.

A truly healthy person must have good health in all three areas: biological, physical, and mental.

Biological

No major or chronic ailments. All organs function properly and normally according to one's age. No need for drugs or supplements to enhance or regulate one's bodily functions. No need for painkillers to ease pains because there is none.

Physical

No disabilities or injuries of any kind and one can perform all the normal tasks without the help of others, special equipment, or medication.

Mental

No psychiatric or psychological problems. One is alert and sociable, optimistic, and happy.

No one is truly healthy, of course. If one were, one wouldn't be able to maintain it forever, for it is inevitable that we, once in a while, will catch some germs, eat the wrong food, get injured, or have unexpected troubles that give us emotional distress. All these could upset our state of health and render us unhealthy until we get rid of them. And, the problem is that we can't avoid them. But, we could deal with them and make them less painful and last shorter. In the following chapters, I'm going to show you how I have dealt with them. Please be reminded that our goal is not to aim at perfect health, but to try to be as healthy as possible.   My *"common sense approach"* is not the only way to do it, and it may not work for you. But, it could help you find your own unique way. Having good health is probably the single most important thing in life because a healthier person generally is a happier person and lives longer, too. Longevity alone, without good health, is not a blessing; it is torture. It only prolongs the suffering. Just pay a visit to any nursing home to see for yourself; you'll know what I mean.

5

How to Attain Good Health

Another misconception people have is that they think attaining good health is a very difficult thing. They think it requires the discipline to stay away from their favorite foods and to stick to the monotonous, tasteless dietary foods, that it requires the determination to sweat and endure the pains of regular and vigorous exercises, and that it requires one to live a dry and mundane life.

It's not true at all! Attaining good health is as easy as *123,* and you don't need to change much in your diet, exercise routine, and lifestyle if you use *good common sense.* Of course, you must have a good diet, a good exercise routine, and a good lifestyle to begin with. If you don't have one yet, don't worry; you can have one easily by making some minor adjustments to cut down on the consumption of unhealthy foods and drinks, to install a regular and effective exercise routine, and to change your harmful lifestyle and negative mental attitude. The key is *moderation, consistency, and patience.* But, you don't have to sacrifice the fun and enjoyment of life in order to attain good health; actually, you'll gain more because you will be healthier, happier, and have more energy to do the things you enjoy doing. There are so many ways to achieve good health, depending on one's general health condition, physical fitness, age, environment, and many other factors. What works for one may not work for others. Everyone is different and we have to find our own ways.

I do not consider myself one of the healthy and long-life people, not yet anyway, for I am only 72 years old, not old enough to be considered a person of longevity. And, I didn't achieve good health until I was 48; only 24 years of good health is not long enough to be credible. But, the way by which I've attained good health is almost exactly how other healthy old folks have attained theirs – using a lot of common sense and self-control. Sharing my personal experiences with you may help you get the same good results.

During my recovery period, I learned a very valuable lesson: don't trust people lightly (including medical doctors) and don't follow others blindly. It's wise to consult as many qualified people as possible but be careful with whom you consult. You definitely don't want to seek medical advice from a lawyer even though he might be a trustworthy old friend. Nor should you ask a person who has no career himself, to help you plan yours. Always pick the one who not only is trustworthy, but also knowledgeable on the subject you are seeking advice on and consult as many of them as possible. Always use *common sense* to evaluate carefully the advice given to you before making your final decision.

In order to attain good health and longevity, I worked on all three areas that I've mentioned above (biological, physical, and mental) simultaneously because they are interrelated and interdependent. The problems of one area may cause problems in other areas. Furthermore, the process of improving health takes time. You must be patient because it takes a long time to realize the good results of hard work and dedication.

6

Biological Health

Among the three, this is the area we have the least control of; it has a lot to do with our DNA, heredity, and luck. If we were lucky, we would be born healthy, with all our body parts functioning normally. That means no defects of any kind, no diseases, and no ailments. If we were not lucky, we would be born with some sort of deformities, abnormalities, or illnesses. In that case, we must seek medical help to correct or cure the problems and, if they can't be cured, we must adjust ourselves and learn how to live with them for the rest of our lives.

Common Sense Approach

That was what I did when I realized, after many years of treatments by numerous doctors and bizarre healers, that my bad hip and general health condition were getting much worse instead of getting better. After thinking logically, I realized that it did not make any sense to continue doing the same thing over and over again. I started to question the logic of our actions. I began to apply the "common sense approach" to solve my problems. I began to *listen* to my body and pay keen attention to the biological, physical, and mental reactions to the foods I put into my mouth, the things I did, and the places I visited.

Listen to Your Body

Probably this is the most important part of the road to good health. It is more important than the regular physical checkup and the blood test because we can perform this function all the time by ourselves and, if anything is wrong with our body, we'll know it before any diagnosis or doctor can tell us. We better use the built-in alarm system that we're born with. It warns us when any part of our body is not functioning properly, from minor headaches due to overwork to repeated dizziness caused by low blood pressure, diabetes, or something else. So, don't ignore the warnings; get medical help as soon as possible. Ignoring repeated warnings definitely will lead to more serious and sometimes irreversible problems down the road.

Our own built-in alarm system is very accurate and reliable compared to the one for our home, it never gives us a false alarm. However, it should not overly alarm us. Minor warnings, such as fatigue due to overwork, pain from over exercise, stomach ache from overeating, and all those non-recurring discomforts of which we know the causes, shouldn't be the reason for rushing to the doctor's office. Let us fix the problems ourselves first. Only those unusual ones that we fail to fix and don't know what the causes are, then, we should take them seriously – go see a doctor or call 911 if you feel your life is at risk.

I always keep a mental record of what I've eaten, where I've been, and what I've done. In case something is wrong, I would have a better idea of the cause of it. Keeping track of our daily activities is very important; if we pay attention to them, they'll tell us in what way each activity has affected our physical and mental wellbeing. If a certain food I ate made me feel good, I'll eat it again to see if it still has the same positive effect on me, the same with exercise and other activities. This good habit remains with me even today when I'm healthy. I *listen* to my body all the time to make sure there is nothing wrong with me. If I should find something that is not quite right, then I'd try to fix it myself first. And, if I can't fix it myself, then I'd go see a doctor. However, I seldom need to see a doctor; I know the causes for most of my problems, and I know how to fix them myself. If I have chest pains after a day of digging and shoveling, I know it's normal and that it is not a heart problem; if my neck hurts and my eyes are tired after watching too much TV or working too long on the computer, then I know I would need to do some stretching exercises or take a walk; or, if my whole body is aching and feeling tired after playing golf consecutively for more than five days, then I know it's time to take a break. Now that I know my body so well, I know how to prevent problems from happening in the first place. Please remember, prevention is always a better option.

After a few years of trial and error and keen observation, I had a pretty good idea of what was good for me and what was not. Vegetables and fruits are friendly to my stomach while deep-fried stuff gives me heartburns, and Mexican and Indian food usually cause indigestion. I've also found out that my personality is my own enemy; being too ambitious and too impatient. I tend to overdo things, and those high jumps and hard running actually hurt my body rather than strengthen it. Even movies and books have certain effects on me. I feel energized and full of hope after watching an inspirational movie in which the underdog becomes a victor by transforming himself through hard work and sufferings. But, a romantic story tends to give me goosebumps because I was brought up in a very strict family; I just can't bear watching two people kissing and fondling without being embarrassed.

In retrospect, listening to my own body probably has saved my life many times over. In one of those times, I caught the flu while visiting my uncle in Macau and did not pay much attention to it until two days later in the middle of the night when I had difficulty breathing. By then, I realized the seriousness of the problem and I called out for help even though I knew it was terrible for me, a guest, to wake up the whole house in the middle of the night and make everybody so nervous. But, when your life is at risk you can't worry too much. Afterwards, at the hospital, I was told that I probably would have died if I had not arrived at the hospital in time. I had pneumonia.

So, please pay attention to your body all the time and listen to what it has to tell you. If anything seems out of ordinary, you should seek medical help immediately to find out what is wrong. It could be something serious. Never ignore the warnings; they may save your life. Many people die unnecessarily because they either don't listen to their bodies or ignore the warnings, construing the red flags as minor discomforts and thinking they'll eventually go away by themselves.

Unfortunately, most people don't listen to their own bodies; taking sex-enhancing drugs is a good example. People should know that erectile dysfunction is a warning sign, telling them that they shouldn't have sex either because they're too old (a natural development) or that they have some kind of biological problems, which would require medical attention. Watching porno movies to stimulate one's sexual desire or taking sex-enhancing drugs to attain an erection is to ignore the warnings. Such acts not only go against nature, but also do a lot of harm to one's body, let alone the danger of side effects caused by the drugs. Another good example of not listening to one's body is to ignore the signs of side effects of the medicine one takes. Even the common over-the-counter remedies have side effects such as heartburn, diarrhea, and allergic reactions.

At the suggestion of a golf friend, I used to take a couple of ibuprofen tablets every time I played golf. It really helped my golf game a lot; my morning stiffness

23

was gone shortly after I took them, and for the whole round I felt energized and played better golf too, because my body was relaxed and loose. But, its effectiveness diminished over time, from six hours to four hours and then to two hours and, therefore, I took more and more of it. It was its addictiveness, however, that frightened me, for I had difficulty quitting it. When I attempted to quit taking it because of the ever-worsening heartburns (one of the side effects of ibuprofen), the pain was unbearable, forcing me to take even more. Realizing the danger of getting hooked and its long-term harmful side effects, I made up my mind to kick the habit. At first it was painful, which made the continuation of taking it much more tempting. But, the stretching exercise came to my rescue. By doing the exercise to loosen up my body before the round, which was not easy to do devotedly at first because it required me getting up an additional half hour earlier, I finally succeeded at kicking the habit. Now I can play golf without pain and without taking any painkillers, and totally avoid all the side effects associated with them. No more heartburn! Of course, my golf game may suffer a little, but I don't care because to me golf is an exercise, not a job.

Drug Abuse

We are a nation of drug addicts; we fall in love with drugs, either illicit drugs, such as heroin, cocaine, and marijuana, or legal (prescription and over the counter) drugs. It is understandable; all our problems will be gone instantly (do they really?) with a few sniffs of cocaine or a few inhales of marijuana and, like magic, all our pains will disappear after swallowing a few tablets of painkillers. It's so easy and convenient that we don't want to spend the time and make the effort to find out the roots of our problems and to have them fixed. It is the quick-fix and instant gratification that make drugs the preferred choice for depression and pain. There are several reasons for the prevailing use of drugs. We're going to skip the illegal drugs and concentrate on the legal drugs only, because the problems with illegal drugs are not what this book is all about. This book is about good health and longevity.

1. It is human nature that we always choose to take the easy way out, getting drunk to forget our problems or taking painkillers to ease our pains. But the easy way is usually the most expensive way and could cost you your life because it is only a bandage approach, curing nothing but delaying proper treatments until it is too late.

2. Our government, which is supposed to protect us, lets pharmaceutical companies brainwash us by permitting them to advertise their products directly to us, on television, in magazines, and on billboards. It also has repeatedly lowered the level of what is considered normal for so many diseases

(diabetes, cholesterol, high blood pressure, etc.), so that many more of us who were considered healthy before, are now unhealthy. And, according to the new standards, many healthy people are led to taking preventative drugs, which are unnecessary. Additionally, they all have serious side effects, but they are huge profit-generators for pharmaceutical companies.

3. Because of the huge profits that can be made, pharmaceutical companies, hospitals, doctors, and retailers all encourage us to consume more drugs. Why should they care? It is our body and our money! Flu shots and vaccines for numerous diseases have become very popular lately even though their effectiveness is minimal, not to mention their long-term side effects, which may not be known until many years later.

4. Because there are many loopholes in our Medicare, Medicaid, and state welfare systems, abuses and frauds are rampant. Doctors prescribe drugs freely because they either want patients to come back often or they are eager to be invited to the all-paid-for and pampering conventions, sponsored by pharmaceutical companies at luxury resorts around the world to introduce their new miracle drugs, which is an excuse for rewarding their most productive doctor-salesmen legally. As a re-

sult, patients are taking more drugs unnecessarily. It is not entirely the doctors' fault though; it is the patients' as well because they can't refuse to accept something that is free. And, there are always some cheaters who falsely claim to be sick in order to get a steady supply of expensive drugs, which they then turn around and sell them in the black markets for profits.

Beware of Drugs

People should know that drugs are not foods; our body has no need for them unless we are sick. They are chemicals, and all have harmful side effects. We should try to avoid them, and if we must take them, then we should be very cautious. Otherwise, we'll have to take more other drugs to counteract the damages done by them, and the vicious cycle continues and turns our body into a battlefield.

Exercising caution with drugs can save us a lot of money, pain, and even our lives. Let me share with you a few true stories to show you how easily one can overlook the dangers of drugs. I have a good friend who had good health all his life until a few years back when he turned 78. We used to play a lot of golf together, and last year, he suddenly couldn't walk without a cane and due to his lack of exercise, he was also overweight. He told me his legs were weak and numb often. When I found out that he had been taking cholesterol drugs (a popular brand which has been heavily promoted), and I had checked out its side effects on the internet, I was convinced that the cholesterol drug he was taking was the culprit of his problems, for one of its side effects had exactly the same symptoms as he had been having. But, when I told him my findings and suggested to him not to take the drug for a while to see what would happen, he was flabbergasted and said, "It can't be! My doctor prescribed it and he should know."

I said, "Yes, he should know, but doctors are humans too; they make mistakes just like you and me. They have so many other patients and so many other things to attend to, there's no way they can care for you as well as you can for yourself. Besides, we're old men now, how many more years we're going to live? The chance of dying from old age is much higher than dying from a heart attack caused by high cholesterol levels. My common-sense reasoning finally convinced him, and he quit taking the drug. Less than a month later, he was back to his old self and never touched the drug again. He is fine now and can still play golf at 83. Another case involves my friend's wife. About ten years ago she had hyperthyroidism and her doctor, young and heavily burdened by mortgage and car payments, was motivated to urge her to have an operation to remove the thyroid. My friend, who has common sense, disagreed because, without her thyroid, she'd have to take thyroid drugs for the rest of her life, which surely will cause other problems in the future. (For sure, the company that makes the thyroid drug would love that; it would have had his wife as a loyal customer for life.) He suspected her doctor was a greedy one who wanted to profit more from the operation. He persuaded her to switch doctors, and she did. Her new doctor didn't think an operation was necessary unless there was no other medicine available to keep her hyperthyroidism under control. She still needs to take thyroid drugs, but she is able to reduce the doses gradually by exercising more and eating well. Now, she is down to taking only one quarter of the medicine her doctor prescribes, and the routine test shows that she is fine. This proves *common sense* does make sense.

My wariness of doctors and drugs came from my own experiences. The first time was the cortisone that put me in the hospital, which nearly killed me. The second time was in 1969 when I went to see a doctor for my bad hip at the clinic of the university I attended. He told me the cartilage of my right hip joint had been badly damaged by arthritis and that there was no cure. The only option was to have a hip replacement, which I couldn't afford at the time. So, he gave me a painkiller with a name so long that I've forgotten how to spell it now. (By the way, it had been banned a long time ago because it was a very potent drug and had numerous and dangerous side effects.) Anyway, it worked wonders for me. My pains were gone like magic, and so was my limping. But, I had to take a blood count test every month to make sure the drug did not have any adverse effect on me. When a pharmacist friend showed me the long list of its side effects, I was shocked. I knew then that it would have killed me if I had continued taking it. I started cutting down on it and took it every other day instead of every day and only took half a pill instead of a whole pill, until I finally quit taking it. For sure, I was miserable at first, but, I was determined to endure the pains and tried to assuage them by doing stretching exercises. Less than a year later, my bad hip still remained the same, but the pains had diminished to the point that they were tolerable due to the combination of stretching exercises and positive thinking. Eventually, I had to have my bad hip replaced, but due to common sense and my caution with drugs, I had avoided the serious damages done to other parts of my body.

More recently, I was diagnosed with diabetes, borderline stage with A1C of 0.65. My doctor put me on medication and instructed me to take the blood test again in three months. I bought the medicine, but after reading the list of its side effects and did some research on the internet, I decided not to obey my doctor, at least for now. I know why my A1C suddenly shot up to 0.65 from my normal of 0.55. It was not that I'm overweight or lack of exercise. My weight is perfect for my age and height, and I have plenty of exercises – golfing, swimming, and walking regularly as well as doing stretching exercises many times a day. It was the indulgent eating that I had had for a few months during which we had many visitors, and I'd spoil myself with all the sweet things they brought as gifts.

Once the root of the problem was pinpointed, I decided to quit eating irresponsibly and go back to my normal diet. As expected, my A1C test three months later dropped slightly to 0.63, which was still higher than my normal, but without medication. My doctor thought that the medication did me good by lowering my blood sugar without any side effects. But, he did not know my disobedience until I made a confession to him three months later when I took another test with even lower 0.62. He is a good doctor though; he did not get upset at my disobedience. He even praised me for doing the right thing.

WARNING

My "common sense approach" is only good for non-emergency situations. When in a life or death situation, we don't have the luxury of choosing among options. We must entrust ourselves to the medical professionals. Most doctors are competent, and most prescription drugs are safe enough. But, we must exercise caution to identify those bad doctors and dangerous drugs. Again, *listen* to your body and use *common sense*. When you feel something is wrong, consult your doctor immediately.

7

Physical Health

This is the area we have the most control of; it is entirely up to us. If we do it right, then we'll have a life-long of good health, providing the other two aspects (biological and mental) are also healthy, of course. If we don't, then we'll get ourselves into the miserable, vicious cycles of drugs mentioned in the previous chapter. Regretfully, most of us don't do it right. Let's not mention those who have low self-esteem and unmotivated bones. But, even for those who are highly motivated, the process of attaining good physical health requires time, knowledge, hard work, and dedication. It's just too difficult for some of us. And, for those aspiring health nuts and dedicated athletes, they usually choose the wrong approach. They are either misled by glamor and fantasies or attracted by thrills. For example, some choose skateboarding, skiing, mountain-biking, football, and other exciting and popular yet dangerous sports, but do not foresee the likelihood of having broken bones, fatal accidents, and lifelong arthritic pains down the road. Also, influenced by the gorgeous bodies on TV, they go to gyms to build bodies so that they can look like a heavy-weight boxer to impress their peers and to win the hearts of their girls. But, they don't know that the poor air quality inside a gym, the straining of their bodies, the supplements they take, and the fatty foods that they eat in order to build muscles as well as the distractions of sexy girls in body-hugging workout outfits, are actually very bad for their health.

However, the worst thing for our physical health is not the polluted air, unhealthy food, contaminated water, sedated lifestyle, over-eating, or even dangerous sports. It is the supplements that greedy merchants push on us. Everywhere you look, there are a myriad of supplements for every imaginable need – from vitamins to muscle and bone builders, and from stimulants to endurance enhancers. The latest fads are energy drinks and bars. They're simply sugary water and candies loaded with caffeine and cheap sugar that sell for ten times the price of the ordinary stuff. Anything you can think of, they have it. Since supplements are not considered prescription drugs, therefore, they are not regulated, and they're highly profitable. Merchants usually display them in the most visible places to attract impulsive consumers, preying on their eagerness to improve their health and performance. And, because they are not regulated, any unscrupulous person can easily get into the supplement manufacturing business. A lot of supplements on the market are downright dangerous – either they are placebos or contain dangerous chemicals. So, next time when you have the urge to purchase supplements, think again, *use common sense!* The best bet is to consult your doctor.

There are three major areas we need to pay attention to in order to achieve good physical health: air quality, water quality, and food quality. We must have good quality for all of them.

Air Quality

Everybody knows that we can't live without air, but not many people are aware of the impacts clean air and dirty air have on our bodies. Ask any auto mechanic, and they can tell you that air filters from cars driven mostly on dirt roads or in the deserts are clogged with dust. Air filters from those driven in the big cities, especially the industrial cities, are clogged with soot. These cars' air filters need to be replaced frequently. Only the suburban cars have much cleaner air filters. Our lungs perform the same way as a car's air filters, but they are not replaceable like air filters. Therefore, we must keep our lungs healthy by breathing clean air. Breathing dirty air will damage them and killing ourselves.

I'm very sensitive to bad air; smoggy air causes my eyes to itch, and chemical fumes make me cough and give me headaches. That's why I avoid going to big cities, avoid following other cars closely, avoid visiting factories, and avoid playing golf on the days they spray fertilizers. I also leave the house for hours the moment the pest control person comes to service our house. That's why I chose to live in the rural area, among avocado and citrus groves, and have hawks, coyotes, squirrels, and roadrunners as my neighbors. There is no noise except for the droning of bees and hummingbirds and the occasional crowing of ravens when they fly into my koi pond for a drink of water, if not hoping to have a fish as a snack. All these eye-pleasing and mind-calming pleasures are nothing in comparison to the air I breathe here though. It is always fresh and scented. Depending on the seasons, I may smell orange blossoms, cherry blossoms, or apple blossoms; I can tell the differences among apricots, persimmons, and avocados just by their fragrances. Sometimes, the air is full of so many different kinds of scents that I have difficulty telling which is which. But, the air here makes me feel good; with every deep breath, I feel every road and river inside me is free of obstacles, and the traffic moves smoothly. With every deep breath, all the pores of my body open up to let in the life-sustaining oxygen. With every deep breath, I feel soothed and relaxed. As we all know, feeling good is very *good* for our body and mind.

Water Quality

Water is another must for us to survive. Good water makes us healthy, and bad water makes us sick. Not like air though, good water is hard to come by. Our city water comes from reservoirs and from rivers hundreds of miles away through aqueducts. It contains numerous minerals (some of them are harmful) and various harmful chemicals. It's undrinkable without water treatment.

Chlorine is added to kill germs and fluoride is added to protect our teeth. Small towns and rural areas get their water from wells, which is not much better because our groundwater is also severely polluted by water runoffs from factories, dairies, and farms. Yes, there are places in this world where we can still have good quality water, but they're either too remote or have temperatures too harsh for humans. Since it's impractical for most of us to move near good water supplies, we have to do the best we can to improve the quality of the water we drink. In my case, I use a soft-water system to cut down a lot of harmful minerals from our city water, and then, I use a reverse osmosis filtration system to filter out more impurities. It's still not perfectly pure, but it is drinkable. To further protect ourselves from bad water, I bring my own water to the restaurant, to the golf course, and always stock a few bottles in my cars.

Food Quality

Like air and water, we must have food to survive. Also, like good air and good water, good food can enhance our health and lengthen our life while bad food can do just the opposite. But, what food is good and what food is bad? Most people think they know. They get their knowledge from the media and from their circles of friends and neighbors. Do they also let the government, the dieticians, or their parents decide for them? Most people do. They *don't use common sense*; they believe what others, especially celebrities and people with a fancy title, tell them. It is amazing that people would drink more coffee, consume more red wine, and eat more chocolate just because they hear it on TV, saying they are good for the body; they would happily spend 30-40% more on food just because they hear it on TV too - that *organic* food is better for you. Or they would stop eating their favorite bread because some dietary gurus say gluten is bad for the body. Have they verified the accuracy and reliability of the sources? Have they ever suspected that they're being fooled by those who could profit from the false statements? Have they ever realized that some foods that are good for others may be bad for them, or vice versa? No, they have not! It is much safer to follow than lead. It's a herd instinct.

Common sense tells me that there are no such things as good foods and bad foods (there are poisonous foods though); there is only good quality or bad quality. All foods can be good or bad depending on *how, how much, when,* and *who* consumes them. To demonstrate my point, I'm going to provide the following examples.

How

We all know that salmon is good for our health (except farmed salmon, which may be raised on feeds containing antibiotics and other poisonous chemicals). But we may get sick if we eat them raw or without proper preparation.

How Much

Although salmon is very nutritious, if we eat too much of it in one meal, we may get sick too. Since our body needs all kinds of nutrients, if we eat too much salmon and not enough other foods to balance it, we may deprive our body of other important nutrients that are vital to our health.

When

It is not only what we eat, but *when* we eat that matters as well. Eating a big breakfast (I don't mean overeating) before a round of golf or before going to work in the fields is much better than eating a light, late dinner right before going to bed because, according to many studies, going to bed with a full stomach is unhealthy.

Who

We all know that red meat and dairy products are rich in protein and fats, which are a good source of energy. They're great for people who engage in demanding physical activities. But, they're very bad for people who are obese and have heart conditions. All foods are not the same; they're different from each other in size, in look, in color, in texture, in taste, and in contents. The vitamins and nutrients they supply are also different. Some are rich in vitamin C and some in vitamin D, some are rich in protein and some in good fats, some are loaded with iron and some with potassium, and the list is endless. In short, all foods are good, and we need all of them. And, we are all different too, so are our needs. Some need more protein, and some need more fats. Some can gain weight easily, and some can eat like a pig and remain thin. That is why we need to listen to our bodies and find out what's good for us and what isn't. Then, we could tailor our diet to eat more of those foods that are good for us and less of those that are not.

Unfortunately, many people are not adventurous; with so many different kinds of foods in this world, they stick only to their old diets (good or bad) and never dare to try something new. It's quite understandable. They are brought up that way, and their digestive systems are accustomed to certain kinds of food. It is not uncommon that some people must have bread, must have rice, or must have noodles. Besides, to try new things is risky; either they don't like them or their digestive systems can't handle them. But, don't let that stop you from exploring. It takes time and patience to change an old habit, the mental attitude, and the digestive system needs to be retrained. (I can eat tons of fruits, but my wife couldn't at first because she'll get diarrhea if she does. But, after gradually adding more fruits to her diet, she can now eat almost as much fruits as I do and without any problems.) This stick-to-the-old habit way of eating is not desirable; one tends to have too much of some nutrients and not enough of others, which *deviates* from the ideal diet.

My family eats almost everything except for those we've tried and don't agree with our digestive systems and for those that are too exotic for our taste. We eat a well-balanced diet; it mainly consists of fresh fruits, seasonal vegetables, and seafood, and a moderate amount of grains and nuts, as well as dairy products and meats. I drink plenty of water, adding fresh lemon juice for flavor and vitamin C. I seldom drink soda pops and prepared juices because they contain too much sugar, preservatives, and other harmful chemicals. However, I do indulge myself once in a while, eating a juicy steak, a cheeseburger, a few slices of pepperoni pizza, or drinking a glass of draft beer or wine. I believe eating should be fun and enjoyable. It is one of those things that we work so hard for, but, like fun and enjoyment, we must do it in *moderation.* Otherwise, it will backfire.

Moderation

Although I eat almost everything, one thing I try very hard not to do is to overeat. Overeating is a prevailing problem in America, and it is one of the major causes of obesity and heart disease besides fatty foods and sugary drinks. It is not that I don't like to eat or have absolute control of my cravings; in fact, my eyes are always bigger than my stomach, and my willpower sometimes goes limp. Only my abhorrence of having a big belly and the apprehension of not being able to hike and play golf are what keeps me sticking to the practice of *moderation.*

(But, what is moderation? Does it have a standard? No. What is moderate for me may not be moderate for you. It depends on our metabolism. Even for the same person, it varies from time to time. Say, a typical lunch of a standard size sandwich and a glass of milk is moderate for a field hand, but an excessive one for a person who sits in the office all day.) But, I do have a practical solution, which makes it easy for me to control myself: I *avoid* temptations. I seldom eat buffets, which is too tempting to overeat. I don't buy and stock up on junk foods at home, but I do stock a variety of fresh fruits and nuts, so more likely, I would have healthy snacks and desserts. Eliminating temptations is the easiest and most effective way of self-control. Moderation is not only a good practice for our eating habits, but also good for every situation in our daily lives. All the healthy elderly people I've interviewed, including my father who lived a healthy life (his psychological sickness aside) all the way to an old age of 93 and probably would still be alive today had he not broken his pelvis, emphasize the importance of moderation for our physical and mental health. Their adages are *to quit eating while you still want more, quit working while you still have some energy left, and quit talking while your audience is still attentive.*

Organic Foods

It's sad that the foods we eat no longer are safe and healthy for our body. Increasingly, farmers use fertilizers to increase yields and pesticides to protect their crops from diseases and pests, and ranchers use hormones and corn to shorten the time needed to get their cattle and chickens to the markets and use antibiotics to reduce the mortality rate. All these chemicals and drugs have been proven very harmful for human consumption. They are the leading causes of many ailments, including cancers. Therefore, some health-conscious consumers (usually more affluent) begin to look for healthier and safer alternatives – organic foods. Organic foods are produce and meats grown or raised with traditional methods, without using artificial fertilizer and pesticide. Small farmers and ranchers, who take advantage of this profitable niche, are happy to meet the demand. As the demand for organic foods grows, more and more big farmers and ranchers jump on the bandwagon, because organic foods generally command higher prices (20 - 50% more) and have higher profit margins. It's inevitable that some unscrupulous farmers, ranchers, distributors, and retailers see the lucrative opportunity. They sell inorganic foods as organic. In the real world, where there's money, there are crooks. It's a shameful truth.

You may argue that organic foods require approval and certification from the FDA, and the rules are strict and clear. But, here again, use some *common sense*! Rules are rules and realities are realities. They are two different things. Does the FDA have enough manpower to monitor the enormous food industry sufficiently? Can it practically enforce its rules? No! Even the IRS doesn't have enough money to hire enough auditors to catch tax evaders; the Justice Department doesn't have the manpower to prosecute Medicare frauds, schemers, and polluters; and the Immigration Department does not have enough agents to defend our borders and, therefore, hordes of illegal aliens and tons of illicit drugs enter this country every day. Do you really think the FDA has the resources and interest to chase after those small harmless cheats who sell inorganic foods as organic? Besides, there are many links in the chain of food distribution – the farmer, the rancher, the distributor, the wholesaler, and the retailer. How would the FDA pin down who is the offender? And, how would it certify imported foods from overseas, where corruption is rampant, supervision is scanty or rules are nonexistent? Sending its agents overseas to make sure foreign farmers and ranchers comply with our rules? Impossible! You may also argue that we can test imported foods for harmful chemicals. But, is it possible to carry out such time-consuming procedures for thousands of containers of foods entering our country every day? Impossible too!

Besides, it's impossible to tell organic from inorganic foods unless you send them to the laboratory for testing. They look the same, smell the same, and taste the same. (Some say organic fruits and produce are usually smaller and not as good-looking and organic chicken is smaller and less meaty. It isn't true. The oranges, avocadoes, peaches, and persimmons I grow organically for our own consumption are just as big and as beautiful as those inorganic fruits on the shelves of the supermarkets. But other fruits, such as apples, cherries, and pears, also grown organically, are disappointments. I think it has to do with climate and soil and many other factors.) And, they don't have individual labels to identify them with. The only option is to trust the merchants. But, can we really trust the merchants with our money? I don't think so because they are in the business to make money. The more the better and selling inorganic food as organic is a lot more profitable.

I don't buy organic foods. It is not because I disagree with the fact that organic food is better for our body than inorganic food, nor do I mind paying a premium for them. I simply don't want to be cheated. There are just too many situations that make me wary of the honesty of food suppliers. Just pay a visit to the supermarket; you'll notice that organic and inorganic fruits and vegetables are displayed side by side (some clever ones may put them in different places), and you can't tell which is which except by the price signs, where the prices for organic items are much higher. But, the funny thing is that the check-out clerks don't know which is which also; they rely on the color of the plastic bag used to bag the things you buy – the green one for organic, and the white one for inorganic. Now, just think, if there were real organic stuff (which should cost more) on the shelves, would they let you have the liberty to choose which colored plastic bag to use? In other words, would they permit you to cheat them? Of course not! They can't be cheated, but you'd be if you're honest enough to use the green bag.

I once asked a foreman, who is in charge of several avocado groves near my house, how they grow organic avocados differently from the inorganic ones. He laughed and said, "We do as we always did, we fertilize the trees through irrigation systems and we spray them with pesticides once a year by helicopters."

"Does any grove here grow organic avocados?" I asked.

"Not that I know. We all sell to the same packing house at the same price."

Obviously, the growers in my area do not sell any of their avocados as organic to the packing house. Who does the cheating then? Someone along the distribution channel, from growers to retailers, must do. I'm not implying that all merchants are cheaters. I'm sure most of them are honest and conscientious, who want to keep us healthy. But, there are some dishonest profiteers out there too, who don't care for anyone else but themselves. But, as a consumer, we don't know what we're buying, organic or inorganic. I wish our government would leave us alone and let us consumers *be aware*! The more it tries to protect us, the more we trust the systems blindly and don't use our heads. The truth is no one in the world can adequately look out for us. We must use common sense and watch out for ourselves.

Farmer's Market

Many people think a farmer's market is a good place to buy organic foods. They believe naïvely that local farmers organically grow the produce, fruits, nuts, and flowers – eggs from the local chicken farms whose chickens are fed only with organic feeds and honey from the local beekeepers whose bees collect nectars *only* from flowers grown without fertilizers and herbicides (they must be very smart bees). People have no idea that most farmer's market hawkers are weekend merchants, and the goods they sell come from wholesalers and local growers, and sometimes from dishonest farm hands who steal from their employers. To believe that the small local farmers follow the FDA's strict guidelines for "organic" labeling, use real organic feeds for their chickens, or that the smart honeybees can distinguish organic flowers from inorganic ones, is ludicrous. It's like the blind leading the blind! Though I like to patronize small local merchants, I prefer not to buy my food from the farmer's market. Besides higher prices, there are other more serious concerns: unlike big, reputable supermarket chains, farmer's market hawkers don't have the manpower nor the resources to ensure the foods they sell are safe for consumption. Their produce and fruits may contain unacceptably high levels of pesticide, and their eggs may be too old or infested with bacteria. Using common sense again, how can their eggs be fresh if they open for business only once a week? What do they do with those unsold eggs?

Moreover, most farmer's market hawkers are transitory merchants, and they are either too small or have too many of them to be inspected by the local health department, much less the FDA. I just feel safer buying from the supermarkets or the reputable neighborhood markets; at least, if there should be anything wrong with their foods, they would have the serial or batch numbers to track them down with and have the resources to notify their customers.

Farm-Raised vs. Wild-Caught

The problem with farm-raised seafood is far more complicated than organic products. Besides the authenticity problem which plagues organic food, farm-raised seafood has another problem: not all farm-raised are bad and not all wild-caught seafood are good. It depends on *where* and *how* they are raised and caught. If they're farmed in clean, natural environments and fed no artificial foods, such as some abalone farms along the isolated coast of California, they are just as good as wild-caught. On the other hand, wild-caught are unsafe for consumption if they're caught in polluted waters such as the Mississippi River, where tons of toxic chemicals are dumped into it from upstream industrial plants along its banks, or along the densely populated coastal areas in Southeast

Asia, where untreated sewage pour into the ocean. Generally, farm-raised seafood is undesirable, because in order to maximize the profit, farmers tend to feed their stocks with hormones and soy to make them grow faster and fatter, as well as with antibiotics to reduce the mortality rate.

I shun buying farm-raised seafood and wild-caught seafood from areas with pollution problems. I prefer deep-sea fish and fish from cold and sparsely populated areas such as Alaska, Argentina, and Chile. I read the labels carefully and prefer U.S.-based companies with the origin of the products coming from the U.S. I have no confidence in foreign companies and foreign products, especially from underdeveloped countries, where there is no official scrutiny, where money is more important than integrity, and where they fake everything, from designer jeans to baby formulas that have killed hundreds of babies. And, I also avoid buying seafood from ethnic markets. They generally have low respect for the laws and the rules, and they make way too many mistakes in labeling – I doubt they aren't intentional – farm-raised often becomes wild-caught and frozen becomes fresh.

I don't buy prepared foods, such as hard-boiled eggs, salads, fruits, and many other conceivable items that have been prepared and packaged in factories for people who are too lazy to boil their own eggs or wash their own vegetables and fruits. (Not that they don't have the time; they have plenty to waste on playing games, watching gossipy news on the Internet, and spending hours each day texting back and forth silly stuff with friends. And yet, they don't have a few minutes to prepare a healthy meal for themselves and for their families.) In order to have prepared foods look fresh and stay tasty, have a longer shelf life and still be price-competitive, harmful preservatives, artificial ingredients, and other chemicals must be used. And, for the same reasons, I avoid canned foods.

My Diet

My current diet evolved from years of good and bad eating experiences as well as advice given to me by healthy old folks. I adopt those foods that do my body good and shun or eat very little of those that don't. It's very simple: I eat everything that is edible (or more fitting, available), and I eat only when I'm hungry. But, I try hard not to overeat or undereat, for I am a true believer behind the philosophy of the creation of "words." The words "over," "under," and "too" have great meanings; they imply "not good," but *moderation* or middle ground is. Although it is hard to apply this simple philosophy to everyday living, I try hard not to do anything *too* much or *too* little.

Breakfast

First thing in the morning, I drink two glasses of warm water to flush my digestive system, eat a plate of fruit (an assortment of avocado, apple, grapes, or berries), a cup of coffee without cream and sugar, a big bowl of oatmeal (briefly boiled with water and also without milk and sugar, but with an egg and a few sprinkles of white pepper), and another cup of warm water to finish off.

Lunch

Unlike breakfast, which is pretty much the same thing, day in and day out, for lunch I eat whatever I want – hamburgers, salads, sandwiches, pizzas, noodles, or what is available at the time. I prefer simple olive oil and dark vinegar in my salads made of as many kinds of vegetables as possible. It doesn't taste as good as other prepared salad dressings (kind of plain), but since I've eaten it this way for a while, I've begun to love it, for it brings out the individual flavor of each ingredient, and it's healthier too. Also, I try to rotate my lunch menu frequently to add variety and reduce boredom.

Snack

Between lunch and dinner, I eat a small cup of plain yogurt with mixed nuts, a banana, or an orange. But, I have to be careful, without discipline and strong willpower, snacks can become full meals, especially with nuts and chips while watching TV or reading a book. To avoid this problem, I take my snack right before I go outside working in my garden for a couple of hours to burn off the calories, so that I won't be able to have more, even if I would want to.

Dinner

Dinner time is about 6:30PM – I try to avoid eating late. Typically, I'd have rice and a soup of mixed vegetables and bones (chicken, pork, or beef bones), slowly cooked for many hours, a vegetable and a meat or fish dish. But, when my wife and I are busy or lazy, we might have a small salad of mixed vegetables and a small steak. Or, even easier, we'd throw in some meats or seafood, vegetables, and tofu, and cook them in a big pot of bone soup (made of bone stocks). We call this kind of cooking "EZpot" because one pot does it all, and it keeps the food warm throughout the course of the dinner. It's great for cold weather, and it's easy and quick, and more importantly, it's healthy. We can have many dinners out of the same pot of soup; all we have to do is to add more things to it. We always have either a glass of wine or a beer with dinner, and a cup of tea afterwards. For dessert, I'd have a piece of dark chocolate, or once in a while, a piece of cake, pie, cookie, or even a scoop of ice cream. But, I never forget to exercise and do other aspects of maintaining my healthy habits.

One habit of mine, I think, contributes to my good health, and that is to take a leisurely walk for at least half an hour after dinner and not eat anything else until the next morning. Since I go to bed late, usually after 11:30, I give myself plenty of time to digest the food, so that I don't have to go to bed with a full stomach. Going to bed feeling full is very bad for our health, according to many studies. It makes us fat because our body, instead of converting the food into energy, stores it as fats. Of course, I feel hungry sometimes when I stay up late, especially after watching those commercials, advertising juicy hamburgers and crispy pizzas. I always have an urge to go down to the kitchen to get myself something to eat. Fortunately, I have good discipline and strong willpower. Resisting temptation is easy for me, anyway. Another habit is that I drink a lot of water throughout the day. I believe, and my doctor agrees, that the benefit of drinking enough water is well worth the trouble and embarrassment of looking for a restroom frequently. Overall, my diet works very well for me, but it may not be for you. Everybody is different. You should do some experiments yourself and make the necessary adjustments to suit your own needs, your schedule, your taste, and your health condition. But remember, to change a bad habit isn't easy; allow some time for the transition and be patient. Good results will come, guaranteed!

My Favorite Foods

As I've mentioned before, I eat everything that is edible, providing that they are healthy foods, but I try to eat in moderation. And I do have certain guidelines to follow if I stay home. But, when we have visitors or when we are traveling, all these good habits and guidelines would be forgotten completely.

Guidelines

1. Food must be fresh. (Check the expiration date and use visual examination.)
2. No harmful chemicals. (No fool-proof way to get around it except to buy from credible retailers and take the chance.)
3. Avoid prepared and canned food. (They are loaded with sodium, saturated fats, artificial colors, preservatives, and other chemicals.)
4. Eat more vegetables and fruits and less meats, especially red meats.
5. Avoid farm-raised seafood. (They are loaded with antibiotics and hormones.)
6. Keep salt, sugar, and fat consumption to a minimum.
7. Avoid eating out. (Generally, restaurant food is not as healthy as home-cooked meals.)
8. Easy to prepare. (Most people don't have much time to cook at home. Be practical and keep it simple.)
9. Economical. (Expensive foods are not necessarily better for us.)
10. Must taste good. If not, who is going to eat it?

My Favorite Dishes

1. Sesame Lemon Chicken --- Easy on sugar, but generous with lemon juice. It may taste a little

sour at first, but it's very good for you. Get used to it.

2. Steamed halibut with ginger, garlic, and green onion.

3. Bake salmon with olive oil and basil.

4. Ground Pork with Black Bean and Water Chestnut and Garlic Sauce --- Don't eat too often because it's fatty.

5. Steamed or boiled vegetables with olive oil --- very healthy and should be eaten more often.

6. EZpot --- Soup of bone stocks with meats, seafood, tofu, and assortments of vegetables. This is my favorite because it's very easy to prepare, relatively inexpensive, highly nutritious, versatile, and all in one big pot. And, it's great for singles because you can get many meals out of one pot. All you have to do is to add more ingredients each time.

My Favorite Desserts

1. Soling's Cake --- Made of all natural ingredients, not too sweet, and not too fatty, but very satisfying, and just perfect.

2. Flaky Egg Tart --- Good but eat no more than two.

Please remember that you don't have to follow my diets and routines exactly; you can eat whatever you like as long as you eat *moderately* and *sensibly*. Don't overeat (remember the 70% rule), and try to eat regularly, for according to the many healthy people I talked to, eating irregularly is not good for you. The reason is clear: our body needs nutrients continuously to provide energy to support various functions and activities. Constant hunger or lengthy hunger could deprive our body of the nutrients it needs. Also, prolonged hunger tends to build up our cravings for food and, when it is available, we are more likely to overeat. By the same token, constant eating and never giving our stomachs a chance to be empty is not good either. The function of our stomachs is to process foods, not to warehouse them. Diversify what you eat – expand your menu and try something new even if you don't like it at first. Sticking to your favorite foods, such as bacon and egg, hamburger, and French fries, and eating them all the time is not healthy eating. Well-balanced meals with many varieties are not only good for our body but also make eating more interesting.

Good Diet and Dieting

Don't be confused with a good diet and dieting. Good diet is eating a well-balanced and the right amount of food that keeps us healthy, and dieting is the way we eat and what we eat for the purpose of losing weight, which isn't necessarily healthy. In fact, most dieting programs do not work; they are get-rich-quick schemes by opportunists who capitalize on the fashionable trend of being slim and thin. Some of them go as far as to use their impressive titles of M.D. and Ph.D. or to employ celebrities as spokesmen to endorse their products or programs. Unfortunately, there are so many people who have a herd mentality problem or are too lazy or lack discipline; they waste money and time and jeopardize their health in believing that they can lose the extra pounds and look great instantly without having to exercise. Sure, taking diet pills and sitting around watching TV are easy. But, they should know that the only way to lose weight naturally and safely is by proper eating and regular exercising, period, and no substitute! Any other ways are temporary fixes and are not long-lasting. Once they quit dieting, the extra pounds they've shed would come back in no time.

Use common sense. How can those prepared meals delivered to your doorsteps once a week and those pills that make you feel full, reduce your appetite, induce vomiting, or diarrhea to get rid of the foods you've just eaten be good for you? They not only deprive your body of the needed nutrition, but also cause unnecessary damage to your body. Even those dieting programs that advocate natural foods (assuming they're true) are not sustainable because they generally lack variety and are thus monotonous. It is difficult to follow them strictly day in and day out; sooner or later, when you become bored with the dietary foods and the craving for your favorite food is strong, you'd be tempted to break the routine, thinking, "Just this one time." But, one time leads to another, and pretty soon you would be back to square one. I don't know anyone who has joined dieting program getting good result.

The Art of Living

People think living well is to live in a luxurious house in an affluent neighborhood, to have expensive cars, to be able to travel around the world and stay at five-star hotels, and to be served and pampered by hordes of people who are fond of your money instead of you. The same kind of thinking applies to eating and drinking. People think going to a five-star restaurant for a five-course dinner of exotic food with fancy plate arrangement while drinking French champagne and expensive wine is eating well and drinking well. Sadly, they miss the boat by miles! I know because I've missed the boat once, too. It took me a long time and quite a bit of money to realize that this kind of living is not living well at all. It is a very unhealthy living. I got fat due to eating too much fatty food, got tired easily due to lack of exercise, and was easily irritated and very unhappy with myself because I got too busy to have time for relaxation. I discovered, fortunately not too late, that to live a simple, carefree life, eat simple food and drink plain water is truly living well.

Living well is an art; it requires learning. Like a wine connoisseur, we need to develop a sense of interest and appreciation for our environment and our food. This applies not only in what we eat, but also in how we eat them – look at them closely to appreciate their shapes and colors, smell them, chew them well to feel their textures, and savor their uniqueness before swallowing them.

When my wife and I first reduced sodium, sugar, and fat in our cooking, the food tasted – what do you think – tasteless. It took us many months to get used to it, and now, we love it because the food actually tastes better without too much salt and grease. We can taste the distinctive flavor of each ingredient when, in the past, we could not. Now, restaurants and prepared food are too salty for us, which is good because we eat a lot less of them. We not only save money, but also eat healthier.

My eating philosophy

Eat what is good for your body first, and then develop a taste for it. Just like marrying a good person first, and then develop love for each other.

Exercise

Good health cannot be attained without regular and proper exercise. By definition, exercise is any activity that requires physical and mental action of employing or putting our body or mind to work. It has no definite forms, and it doesn't require a specific time or place or special equipment. We can exercise anytime, anywhere, and with whatever we have – from strenuous sports to leisure-walking, from weightlifting in the gym to riding a stationary bicycle at home, or from just simply rotating our tired necks at the desk while we're working on the computer. To exercise our brain, we can count, do jigsaw puzzles, play poker, or simply daydream. But, for more intensive mental exercises, I prefer to socialize, share jokes, or even engage in friendly arguments.

Every part of our body, including internal organs and the brain, are built to be used and perform certain functions. Like engine parts, they would become rusty if they are not used, worn out if they are overused, subjected to abusive use, or used without proper maintenance. Therefore, we must exercise our limbs properly and regularly by moving, our lungs by breathing, and our brains by thinking and so on. We also must maintain our body parts properly and regularly by providing them with the right kind of nutrients and the right amount of time to rest.

Exercise, however, if not done correctly, can do more harm than good. Many people think going to the gym and hiring a trainer to build a gorgeous looking body are good for their health, but, from my own experiences, it is quite the contrary. For one thing, the gym is not an ideal place to exercise; it's too noisy and has too many distractions for it to be a relaxing environment to rejuvenate our mind and body. Secondly, most trainers are so wrapped up in muscle-building that they generally overlook the need to design a program to fit an individual. In my case, even with my telling him that I'm old and what I want is to maintain my current physical health, I still ended up, after only three sessions, with my feet injured due to aggressive training. I don't mean that we shouldn't go to the gyms at all; I regularly go to the hotel gyms to have a quick session of exercise when I travel, because they're better alternatives than jogging in busy and smoggy streets or walking in an unsafe neighborhood.

Set a Plan

Work out an exercise plan according to your age and health condition. Even if you're young and healthy, you should avoid those strenuous exercises that could cause injuries because, once you're injured, it is hard to maintain good health again due to the fact that you'd have to take painkillers to ease the pains, which may also forbid you to exercise. After age 40, you should choose those exercises that would increase flexibility, enhance balance, and strengthen your heart. Flexibility and good balance help reduce the chance of injuries, and a good heart is a sure way to live longer.

Moderation and Consistency

Most people, especially those who are highly motivated, violate the "moderation" rule. They over-exercise. They want to see results right now and don't have the patience to achieve their goals slowly. On the opposite end, those who are less driven violate the "consistency" rule. They either give up easily or are too lazy to stick to their routines. They exercise sporadically, depending on their moods. Either way is not good. In order to get good results from exercise, one must do it *moderately* and *consistently*. Moderation reduces the chance of injury, and consistency improves your health slowly, but surely. Again, as in eating, moderation in exercise varies from person to person and from time to time. A round of morning golf, 45 minutes of afternoon up-hill-and-down-hill walk, and two 20-minute sessions of stretching exercise are enough for a healthy old man like me, but they aren't enough for a healthy young man and are too much for a person who is out of shape. So listen to your body; it will tell you the right amount of exercises you need – if you feel tired and have pains afterward, then you are probably over-exercised. Also, similar to eating, I believe we can get more benefits out of exercises by simply rotating the physical and mental exercises – doing short sessions of stretching exercise in between sedentary activities, such as reading, watching television, and doing computer works. That way, we can balance the two activities of different natures – one is to exercise the body, and the other is to keep the brain active. Additionally, boredom and fatigue caused by engaging in one activity for too long can be avoided.

Make Exercise Fun and Easy

It's easy to set a goal and devise a plan, but, like New Year's resolutions, it's not so easy to stick to it. When the impulse is gone and the excitement wears thin, then exercise becomes boring. And, when this happens, it's impossible to make it a part of our daily routine. That's the primary reason most New Year's resolutions fail because they're too ambitious and too demanding. To turn exercise into a habit, it must be fun, must be a game, must provide plenty of challenges through competition, and most importantly, it must be affordable, accessible, and easy to learn. It is no surprise that soccer, basketball, and table tennis are far more popular than golf and skiing worldwide. All we need is a ball, and we can play almost anywhere and anytime.

No Hobby no Retirement

If you don't have any hobbies by the time you're ready to retire, don't retire! Keep on working as long as you can until you find at least one. If you must retire from your regular job, find another one (a part-time or a volunteer job may do). You must have something to do to keep you busy. I don't have to tell you how many retirees die within a few years after retirement. They die of boredom and sedentariness. Find yourself at least one hobby or develop one if you don't have one yet. Most people treat exercise routines as a leisure activity, like a picnic, a BBQ party, or a walk on the beach. They do it only when they have the time and are in the right mood. But, to make the exercise routine effective and achieve the results it intends, we must make time for it and do it no matter if it's rain or shine. Treat it like a job on which our health depends.

My Exercise Routine

Like my diet, it evolved over time from personal experiences and advice from healthy old folks. I always copy what others do that appeal to me. I'd give them a try to see if they benefit me. The stretching exercises that have helped me a lot came from a golf buddy. When we shared a motel room together at a golf tournament a long time ago, I saw that the first thing after he got up was to spend a half hour on the floor doing them. He told me that he had been doing that since he could remember. Because he was 65 and in excellent shape, I needed no further encouragement; I made his stretching exercises as part of my daily routine ever since.

I golf four to five times a week in the early mornings, walk 45 minutes almost every afternoon up and down my long and hilly driveway, climb an average of 500 steps a day at home, and in between, when I feel stiff, I'd add a few fifteen-minute stretching exercises. In the summer when the days are warmer and longer, I swim several times a week. When I golf, I seldom drive; I let someone else do the driving so that I have more opportunities to walk. I also do deep breathing a lot during the round, like a turbocharger of a car's engine; it not only relaxes me, but also gives me more power. Golfing gives me the combined benefits of exercise and relaxation and, at the same time, allows me to act and laugh like a silly kid again without worrying about being ridiculed. Walking the hilly driveway is for my heart, and the stretching exercise is for my flexibility and balance. Other chores such as gardening, car-washing, fruit-picking, and tree-trimming are vigorous enough to keep my muscles in shape. But, I think stretching exercise is the most beneficial for older folks, for it doesn't require much strength and has less chance for injury.

I've been following my exercise routine for more than 15 years now, and I'm clearly getting good results out of it. At 72, I'm thin and have no belly. I seem to have as much energy as when I was fifty years old despite my ears not being as sharp and my memory not as good anymore. And, I have no pain or ailment of any kind, and I don't need to take any medicine. Compared to friends my age, I look much younger. In the winter, I wear short-sleeved golf shirts while they have to wear a sweater or a jacket. I can hike for hours in rough terrains while they can barely walk without a cane. I can work under the blazing sun for a whole day, pulling weeds and pruning trees, which they consider impossible.

The other day we had a discussion among us healthy golfers about the physical differences between Asians and Westerners. When young, Asian men and women look younger than Westerners, but after sixty and older, they obviously look older. One of the reasons, we concluded, is that elderly Westerners are generally richer, eat better, and stay active longer. They have more hobbies and social life and still participate in sports while most elderly Asians confine themselves to home, living an inactive life. Another reason is that in general Western seniors are more financially secure because they have social security and Medicare and, therefore, they have better health care.

My Stretching Exercises

To me, this is the most important part of my exercise routine. Partly because I have arthritis and partly because it's hereditary, I have a hard time keeping my back straight. My father and my older brother had hunched backs after fifty, and a nephew and a niece became stooped in their teens. I'm sure I would have followed the same path if it were not for the stretching exercises. They help me in two ways: one is to keep my bones and joints healthy and flexible; the other is to remind me all the time to keep my posture erect. I'm not perfectly straight, however, and my body is more rigid than a normal person's. The damage had been done a long time ago by arthritis. But, at least, the stretching exercise has effectively halted further damages and enabled me to function as a normal person again. Again, my stretching exercises might not be suitable for those of you who don't have my problems. I suggest you consult your doctor and your trainer to help you design an exercise routine that is compatible with your age and health condition. Once you have an exercise routine, you must stick to it and follow the "moderation" and "consistency" rules.

Stand-Up Exercises

1. Touch Toes --- Bend forward (breathe out) and try to touch your toes with your fingers, and then straighten up (breathe in) all the way until you bend backwards.
2. Squatting --- Stand straight and lower your body (breathe out) to a squatting position and stand straight (breathe in) again.
3. Horizontal 90-Degree Turn --- Stretch out your arms and make a 90-degree turn to the left and then to the right.
4. Vertical 90-Degree Turn --- The same thing except swing the hands up and down instead of left and right.
5. One Leg Stand --- Stand on one leg and hold the other foot with a hand and try to straighten your spine at the same time.

Lie-Down Exercises

1. Touch Toes --- Bend forward (breathe out) and try to touch your toes with your fingers, and then straighten up (breathe in) all the way until you bend backwards.
2. Nodding Neck --- Lie flat on your back and let your head rest on the palms of your hands. Raise your head (breathe out) and lower your head (breathe in).

3. Upper Body Turn --- Lie flat on your back and let your head rest on the palms of your hands and bend your legs. Turn your body to the right (breathe out), and then return to the previous position (breathe in). Do the same on the left side.

4. Raise Buttock --- Lie flat on your back, hands on the floor, bend your legs, and raise your buttocks (breathe in). Then, slowly lower them (breathe out). Make sure you feel your spine pressed against the floor.

5. Whole Body Stretch --- Lie flat on your back and feel your spine and neck pressed against the floor and hold them there. Fully stretch your legs and arms (breathe in) to feel the toes and fingertips reach out in the opposite direction. Then, swing your arms back (breathe out) to touch your thighs and, at the same time, arch your back ankles towards the torso.

6. Open Up --- Lie flat on your back and let your head rest on the palms of your hands and bend your legs. Slowly open up your arms and legs (breathe in) and try to make your elbows and knees touch the floor. Then, go back to the previous position (breathe out).

7. Raise Legs --- Lie flat on your back and hands on the floor. Raise your right leg (breathe in) as high as possible, and then lower it down (breathe out). Do the same with your left leg.

8. Cycling --- Lie flat on your back, hands on the floor, and start circling your legs in the air.
9. Half Sit-Up --- Lie flat on your back and let your head rest on the palms of your hands. Slowly raise your head and your feet, and at the same time put them down slowly.
10. Deep Chest Breathing --- Breathe in slowly and deeply to fill the whole lung and breathe out slowly to empty the lung.
11. Deep Stomach Breathing --- The same thing, except, fill and empty the stomach instead.

I always finish my stretching routine with the Deep-breathing exercises, because by then, my body is so relaxed and my mind so calm that I routinely fall into deep sleep. It is not a long sleep, only about fifteen minutes long, but it's the most rejuvenating sleep. To achieve this wonderful phenomenon, I have to block out all other thoughts and try to do it very slowly and relaxingly as if I had all the time in the world, so that I can concentrate on the feelings of each movement of my body.

8

Mental Health

Probably mental health is the most important of all three, for biological and physical health are greatly affected by the health condition of our mind. Generally, pessimistic, unhappy, or angry people are more vulnerable to other health problems, such as high blood pressure, diabetes, paranoia, insomnia, and eating disorders. They're apathetic to exercise and sports, dislike socializing with other people and, consequently, they become victims of depression and obesity. In short, they're unhealthy people.

On the other hand, happy people are usually healthier. They have more fun and have more friends, and they are very active. You may argue that happiness won't make a person healthy; he is happy because he is healthy and has no illness. You might be right. It's a chicken-and-egg situation, and no one knows for sure the answer. But, whatever the answer is, it's irrelevant, for we're here to discuss how to achieve good mental health.

Happiness

Happiness is a manifestation of good mental health, and it is a mental state of wellbeing. A happy person feels good about himself and the people around him, and he's optimistic about the future. Feeling good is unquestionably good for our health – many clinical studies have already demonstrated this point. But, how do we keep ourselves happy when there are all sorts of problems in this world – if they're not our own, they're our family's, our friend's, our neighbor's, our country's, or even the world's? Well, there are many ways to minimize if not totally eliminate these problems that bother us if we use common sense, but the most effective way is *to play game* with ourselves. It is a mind game of looking back at our present problems from a perspective of years later in the future. You will be surprised by the difference in feelings, from painful of now to the indifferent of the future.

Be Content

Never ever compare with other people for whatever reason because we're all very much different from each other, which not only makes comparison difficult and unfair, but also meaningless. Keeping-up-with-the-Jones is a sure way to lead us to misery, because should we keep up with one Jones, there will always be another and the keep-up will never end. This doesn't mean that we shouldn't have dreams, shouldn't have ambitions, and shouldn't have desires. Oh, yes, we can have all these and still can be content. You may want to ask: "How can we be content if we don't get what we want, and our dreams unfulfilled?" Yes, you can if you think this way: "It's not my turn yet, and mine will come sooner or later," or "Well, I've tried my best." From a more practical point of view, it is impossible to have all our dreams come true, and all our wants fulfilled. We should be very happy that we have the opportunity and have the courage to give it a try. Of course, you may say these are only excuses to fool ourselves. But, does it matter if they help keep us happy?

Stress Control

No one lives a stress-free life, probably not even a Saint. Life is full of stresses; they come from sickness, family, business, occupation, and even from sports and games. I know a golfer who couldn't get his ball out of the sand trap, and he was so stressed that he had a heart attack and died. There was also an old man who died at the poker table after he won a big pot with a full house. I have many workaholic friends who wouldn't take it easy until after they had a wakeup call – a heart attack or a stroke that put them in the hospital. I told them to slow down, but they gave me all kinds of excuses. "I've got a lot to do," they said, "I must finish this by tomorrow and I have to do it myself for this is a very important project."

Well, I understand because I was like them when I was young. I didn't think I would ever get sick, let alone die from working, and I didn't trust that anyone could do a better job than I could. I thought of myself as indispensable. Not until I'd seen enough people I knew who had heart surgeries or died of heart attacks (and myself having chest pains occasionally) did I realize that I must change the way I work, or I could end up like them.

At first, I walked away from whatever I was doing, even if it were an important meeting when I felt the chest pain was coming – a compressing sensation – and took a slow walk outside the office until the familiar sensation was gone. But, I knew this was not a long-term solution because the frequency of my chest pain increased over time, and it also took a longer time to go away. Sometimes I had to spend hours in the park just to get rid of it. I was quite sure what caused my chest pains; it was the stress from working long hours and the pressures of meeting deadlines, for they occurred mostly in the late afternoons when I was tired, and the anxiety of going home to my family before dark was at its peak.

"What a fool you are," I scolded myself. "If you keep on working like this, you won't live long enough to enjoy the fruit of your labor, and you'll bring misery to your family."

"But, I have so much to do and nobody can do it for me. It's only temporary; when I make a little more money, I'll hire more employees, and then I can relax." I made all the excuses that I could think of.

"That's not true. You think you're the best, and you think you're Mr. Indispensable! What's wrong with you? You've got an MBA and were trained to manage other people. Now, you're working yourself to death! Is the world going to stop if you were sick or dead? Nobody is indispensable, you fool!"

My self-examination woke me up; it reminded me that nothing in the world was worth more than my health, and I'm not doing my family any favor if I don't take care of myself. I made it a routine to leave the office at three o'clock to pick up my two children from school and go play golf with them, in order to avoid the two most stressful hours that routinely gave me chest pain. The prevention strategy proved very effective; by preventing the chest pains, I actually made them disappear. I have had no more chest pains ever since. But there are other more acute stresses, such as chronic illness, accident, death of a family member, divorce, business failure, etc., which are so traumatic and so emotionally charged that they're not easily kept under control. We all know that when we're sober and clear-headed, we shouldn't cry over them because crying and being sad won't help anything. Common sense tells us that we must be *positive* and *optimistic* in such a dreadful time. But, it is very difficult to do because we all have emotions, and emotions take courage and determination to overcome.

I know because I've been there many times before. During those years when I was sick, I was so depressed and withdrawn that I almost cut off all of my social contacts. When I was refused a visa to go to America to study, I was so upset that I downed half a bottle of whisky. When I thought I had lost my love, I was so sad and hopeless that the idea of committing suicide went through my head several times. And, when I was flat broke after losing all my money on my dream project of starting a chain of Chinese restaurants, ignoring the advice of my father, I was so ashamed of my failure and so mad with myself that I couldn't face him for years.

One Sunday morning in February 1992, after being informed by an employee of mine that the area where my office was located had been flooded due to heavy rainfalls for a week, I went to the office with my family to examine the situation. Due to the parking lot being covered with foot-deep muds, I left my family inside the car and went into the building by myself. After opening the door with much difficulty, because of all the mud behind it, I saw 4-foot-high water marks on the walls. Peeping through the opening to the warehouse, I saw boxes of video tapes, which had been stacked up neatly on pallets, were now scattered around on the floor like debris after a hurricane. More than a quarter of a million dollars of inventory was totally destroyed – a total loss and no flood insurance! I don't remember what went through my mind and what my feelings were at that moment, and even today, I still don't understand how I was able to be so cool and calm. But, I do remember that I closed the door and went back to the car and said to my wife and my two kids as though nothing had ever happened, "It's all right, let's go have breakfast at Swing Inn." After all, it was Chinese

New Year Day, and it should be a very happy day; it happens only once a year and, traditionally, we are supposed to celebrate with families and friends. The problem could wait, I thought.

There is one plausible explanation that I can think of for my calmness. I'd failed so many times in the past, and every time I failed, I was able to bounce back higher and stronger than before, which gave me the confidence to believe that this time would be no different. Experience had taught me how to play tricks on myself; I would imagine myself four or five years into the future and look back at the present situation. This way, I was able to detach myself from the emotional factors and enable me to look at things from a more logical and sensible perspective. I'm sure everybody has a few dark moments in his life, which have caused pains, heartbreaks, and despairs. But, these dark moments are no worse than old wounds after they are healed – they can't hurt any more. Looking back at those old miseries, which had hurt so much then, are now only memories, evoking nothing more than a good laugh. I taught my trick to quite a few friends to help them get out of their misery, but most of them simply couldn't duplicate my success even though they tried and knew it was a sensible thing to do. Like quitting smoking, drinking, or doing drugs, it's easy for some, but almost impossible for others, depending on the willpower of the individual. Willpower is not born with, we can acquire it through training or through personal experience.

There are basically two ways of stress control: the Western way and the Asian way. The Western way is to release it by getting angry, yelling, and screaming, throwing, and kicking things. The Asian way is by practicing either tolerance or submission. They blame their misfortunes on fate and accept them, and if they can't accept them, then they tolerate and suffer silently. I don't agree with either way; both ways are temporary fixes. Getting angry is showing excessive emotion, which does not solve any problems, but rather aggravates them. Your anger will cause other people to get angry, and their anger will further irritate you. The Asian way of tolerance is no better because, like the Western way, the roots of the problems remain unresolved. Outwardly, you may look calm and at ease, but inside, your stress is building up silently like a time bomb waiting to explode. My way, playing psychological tricks on ourselves is a more logical solution to our problems; it fundamentally changes the way we look at and react to our miseries. True, it may still not solve any problems, but at least, it helps us get out of depression and into a more positive mood so that we can devote more time and energy to deal with the real problems at hand.

Letting Go

Another way to reduce stress is to let go. Don't be confused though; to "let go" and to "give-up" is not the same thing. To "give-up" is a concession with unpleasant feelings and to "let go" is a concession without the bitter feeling that makes you unhappy. Everybody knows to "let go" is a good thing and is necessary as a way of relieving stress. But, how many people can really let go – I mean truly let go? Not many! It takes understanding, practice, experience, and of course, a lot of time to master this useful practice. But, I've learned a few things through the years that make "let go" a lot easier. I simply say: "I've tried my best and there's nothing more I can do." It's much easier when you've fulfilled your responsibility and don't have a guilty conscience.

Meditation

While to "let go" is passive (you react to something that has already happened), meditation is proactive (you act to prevent something from happening). Meditation, which is a daily routine for monks and nuns, now becomes very fashionable, is a very effective way of relieving stress and attaining relaxation once you've mastered the technique. But, to master the technique is not easy; it requires patience, a lot of practice, and a quiet place away from distractions. For that reason, it is nearly impossible for an ordinary person to adopt it into his daily life, for he just doesn't have the luxury of finding the time and a quiet place for it. Mindfulness is a trendy version of meditation, which is an old body in a new hat designed by opportunists to sell more books and programs. It is used to attract those who have the penchants for fashion. But, there are many other ways to attain relaxation and peace of mind without going through the hassles of meditation or mindfulness, and we can practice them at any time and in any place. All we need to do is put our minds into whatever we're doing at the time and enjoy the process. Smelling the flowers while taking a walk or tending to our gardens, watching the movements of ants and caterpillars while sitting under a tree, appreciating the changing colors of the sky at dawn or sunset, or just listening and feeling the breeze caress our faces, are some of the things we can do easily to relieve stress.

For the same reasons as going to the gyms to exercise, I consider spending our precious time on meditation or mindfulness is wasteful. We can reap the same benefits from performing so many productive activities if we can concentrate only on what we are doing at the time and nothing else. For me, they're golfing, hiking, swimming, gardening, and even doing minor repairs. I know golfing, hiking, and swimming are not exactly as productive as gardening and fixing things, but at least, I have one more thing than meditation, which is exercise.

I doubt how many people who practice meditation truly master the technique and benefit from it. They're more likely to do it out of vanity, differentiating themselves from their more humble and ordinary friends, just like acquiring a new car to make a statement. I know many of my friends and I can't do meditation. I built a meditation room when I built my house, which was the exact copy of the one I had seen in Japan, complete with the raised tatami floor, meditation cushions, and four empty white walls. The only thing in the room is a life-size brush painting of Buddha himself in a meditative posture. I have tried to sit and imitate, but it doesn't work for me! As soon as I close my eyes, Buddha disappears and all the colorful fantasies of the world appear on the wall in front of me. All those things that I'd tried so hard to get rid of would come back to fill my head. Now, the cool and quiet meditation room is another storage room, and the meditation cushions are not seated by me but by piles of old toys.

I'm not saying you shouldn't go to the gym or practice meditation or mindfulness. If you think they've helped you to relax, then, by all means, continue to do it. But, they are not for me. Nor are they for most of the healthy old folks I've interviewed. They are more like me in that they have always managed to relax while they're doing what they enjoy doing.

Psychological Sickness

One of the symptoms of poor mental health is psychological sickness. Unlike real sickness, this kind of sickness is not sickness at all. It is an imaginary sickness created in one's mind, and the only cure is also one's mind. The mind, like a switch, can turn the sickness on and off at will; but a sick mind needs to be fixed before it can turn off the imaginary sickness.

There is no lack of people I know who suffer from psychological illnesses, and I am sure you know quite a few too. My aunt and my father, whom I know very well, are excellent examples. They were sick a lot for most of their adult life – not serious sickness, but minor discomforts here and there. The only times when they didn't feel sick were, for my aunt, playing Mah-jongg and for my father, chattering with friends or hiking in the mountains. Whenever my aunt claimed she was sick, her husband would invite her Mah-jongg friends to come over to their house to play a game with her, and then, her sickness would disappear long before the game would end. My father's sickness would also disappear before the placebo pills, prescribed by his doctor, hit the bottom of his stomach. He unnecessarily spent quite a bit of money on doctors and medicine. Nevertheless, they both lived a long life; my aunt was 94 and my father, 92, when they died.

Although they did not lead a happy life as they should have because they were sick most of the time, their psychological illnesses, I suspect, actually contributed to their long life. They both were hypochondriacs and had false alarms frequently, which compelled them to see a doctor and have another round of physical examination. It's not necessary most of the time, but occasionally, they did find some minor problems and got them fixed early before they would cause serious damages. Just like a car, if you notice a minor problem early on and get it fixed, you may prevent costly repairs or a deadly accident.

Even I, whom I believe to have a sound mind and a lot of experiences in dealing with sickness, could be a victim of psychological sickness. It was three years ago when my wife measured my blood pressure after she had measured hers. It was 117 and 66 – low but quite normal for me. But, my pulse of 49 shocked her, and she cried aloud, "Oh, too low! You'll have a sudden death."

"What's sudden death?" I was alarmed, too, as I heard the word "death."

"Sudden death is when your pulse is too low; you may die suddenly in sleep."

I was speechless, for my wife is medically savvy even though she is not a medical doctor. She was forced to learn all these medical stuff throughout the years, taking care of our two children full-time. She is a quasi-doctor in our family, and her opinion carries some weight. Not a particularly nervous person, I had always been unusually calm, logical, and not easily scared of anything, but this time was different. Almost immediately, I felt I was short of breath when I spoke after our daily 45-minute walk, and I felt I was going to faint when I got up from crouching. In short, all of a sudden, I felt all the symptoms of a weak heart, which I had never felt before. Stressful emotions immediately took over, and the dread of an imminent heart failure entered my head, and all the logical deductions of facts and evidence failed to convince me that I was sound and well.

Without delay, I went to see my doctor who measured my blood pressure, listened to my heartbeats, and had the nurse hook up an EKG monitor to my chest. As he suspected and, to my incredulity, he told me the next day I was fine. When I asked him why my pulse was so slow, he said that I have an athletic heart, which is a powerful heart, like a V-8 engine, that would last for a long time. I left his office feeling better, but not without skepticism. I had no confidence in his diagnosis because he is a general practitioner and not a heart specialist.

The shadow of "sudden death" still lingered in my head, and I still felt some of the worrisome symptoms of heart disease occasionally. I decided to go to a heart specialist to make sure, once and for all, that my heart is okay. I went to one of the best clinics in San Diego. Again, they measured my blood pressure, listened to my heartbeats, and hooked me up to an EKG monitor for 24 hours. The next day when I came back, they gave me a treadmill test. The nurse stopped me after I had finished level 5, and she said, "That's enough, you did great. Most patients who took this test couldn't go past level 3." When the cardiologist, after having reviewed all the reports, told me, "Your heart is fine and you'll live forever," I was absolutely relieved. I floated out of his office 100 pounds lighter.

More recently, my wife experienced pretty much the same psychological problem as I had, except hers was more acute. She has had high blood pressure for years, and she is able to keep it under control with medication. But, every time she has her blood pressure checked at the doctor's office, it is much, much higher than normal. Her doctor told her jokingly that she has "white coat syndrome." Things changed for the worse last year when a few friends and relatives died of heart attacks or became incapacitated by strokes. They all had high blood pressure. Perhaps, because of the traumas of losing so many loved ones in such a short time and the sudden awareness of the grim prospect of having high blood pressure, my wife became increasingly edgy. At times, she was downright paranoid when her blood pressure was higher than normal and wanted me to take her to the hospital right away.

At first, I was able to calm her down with logical reasoning – to convince her that her heart was fine because her daily blood pressure measurements taken at home were normal, that she still could walk our steep and long driveway for 45 minutes without difficulty, and that she never had heart problems before. Her problem was a psychological one, and she knew it, too. But as her problem progressed, logical reasoning failed to calm her. Frequently, and without any particular reason, her blood pressure would shoot up, followed by her pounding heart. She knew that all these were self-made, but she could not help it. In order to solve her psychological problems, I persuaded her to have a thorough heart checkup with a cardiologist, just like the one I had a few years back. And, that did it. After the specialist declared her heart was healthy, all her imaginary problems were gone and never returned since.

These examples demonstrate how important our minds are to our overall health. They could cause more problems than the biological and physical aspects of our body could, and they are much more difficult to detect and cure. Most of us do not even know we have psychological problems, and even if we do know, we are reluctant to admit it, for the word "mental illness" is a scary one, and nobody wants any part of it. But, everybody has it, more or less. So, don't be embarrassed to get help if you cannot deal with it yourself, and pay more attention to your mind by making it knowledgeable, logical, and strong.

Keep the Mind Young

We all know a young mind can help us stay young and healthy and being surrounded by young people is the best way to keep our mind young. It is the natural way, and it's very logical in the old days, when multi-generations living together was the norm. Grandparents take care of the grandchildren while the young adults work in the fields. This is a great arrangement; young children have someone loving and caring to take care of them, and the old have innocent children to keep them active and happy. Taking care of a young child requires constant movements, and an innocent child has the natural ability to make even a sad person happy. That is why old people living with grandchildren are generally healthier.

But in our modern society, multi-generation living arrangement is a rarity, especially in developed countries where most people are financially independent or have social and governmental assistance. Besides, young people these days prefer not to live with their parents and like to raise the children their own ways – with the help of nannies or daycare centers. For those who can't afford such services and are forced to ask their parents to take care of their kids, they seldom give them the freedom as to how to raise their children. Therefore, it could be a very stressful situation for grandparents because they are afraid to discipline their grandchildren even though they think their bad behaviors warrant it.

We can, however, still have the benefit of multi-generation living without actually living with our children and grandchildren; we can spend more time at the parks where children play. Although they are not our own, the end result is almost the same and without the burdens and responsibilities that come with child rearing. We'll feel like kids again just by watching the innocent children play; their energy and playfulness are infectious. But, I don't believe in the idea of having a young wife or a young girlfriend to improve one's health and longevity as many men think it would; it is only a selfish, chauvinistic excuse. According to history, most Chinese kings, who could have as many young wives as he desired, had poor health, and died young, which is a credible proof that confirms my thinking. But, I do believe that monks and nuns have a better chance of leading a healthier and longer life than us ordinary folks, and the reason is clear: they're vegetarians and exercise regularly, and more importantly, the normally remote and isolated locations of their temples provide the perfectly healthy environments – fresh air, pure water, organic vegetables, and no stresses associated with having families, relatives, and friends, enabling them to live a carefree lifestyle, yet with group supports.

The idea of living in a retirement community, thinking the association with people of the same age would better suit us, couldn't be more wrong. It is true that such a place usually has luxury facilities – a golf course, swimming pool, game room, and ballroom – which most retirees can ill afford, and the opportunities to participate in many social functions and activities are endless. But, these benefits were more than offset by the lifeless and depressing atmosphere – visiting the sick at hospitals and going to funerals become a daily routine and talking endlessly about health problems and medicines dominate their conversations. The decaying scene at the cafeteria where lonely, old people munch on their food quietly, and the depressing topics of social and political issues on which they express their opinionated judgments, could make even a young person feel old instantly. However, for lonely, old folks without families and friends or whose families and friends have forgotten about them the moment they become old, sick, and poor, senior citizen communities, or even nursing homes, may be a better option.

9

Fate

Fate is what we commonly call "luck" or, statistically, "probability." It is an elusive thing, which we can't explain and have no control of. No matter how diligently we do all the right things to be healthy and live a long life, there is no guarantee that we will make it; we could get sick or die young all the same if our fate is against us. There are so many factors that are out of our control and can affect our health and longevity.

Since we have to eat, drink, breathe, and go places, there is no way for us to control the quality of air, water, and foods – let alone accidents, wars, natural disasters, and epidemics. If we are unlucky, any one of these out-of-our-control things could happen to us. I'm sure among the people you know, there are quite a few who have tragic car accidents, develop cancers out of nowhere, or get shot by a sniper while cruising on the freeway going to work. And, many more get sick, go broke, and have a divorce as well as other life-changing problems.

It's true that even if I want to eat the right foods and do the right things, I still may not be able to live a healthy life. When we travel abroad, we still have to eat those fruits and vegetables grown in foreign countries, which might contain more harmful chemicals than those grown at home because of the lax regulations. We still have to drink their water and breathe their air no matter how dirty they are. We still have to go places and meet people where we could easily catch germs and get sick. Even if we stay at home and don't travel, we still have to eat at restaurants occasionally and buy foreign fruits and vegetables when local supplies are not available.

That doesn't mean we should give up doing the right things and indulge ourselves doing all the wrong things though. We should try our best to live a healthy and productive, long life and leave the rest to fate. We want to live a healthy and long life because we want to enjoy life more, be able to do all the things that make us happy and fulfilled, and to have more time to do them. It is absolutely not the other way around: to live a healthy and long life just for the sake of having good health and longevity. We must strike a balance: to enjoy life and also to do all those right things that could help us achieve good health and longevity. After all, life without good health can't be enjoyable; it's a miserable life. On the other hand, life without enjoyment and fun is not life at all.

Many people don't even try; they give up because, to indulge in foods, drinks, and other pleasures, is a lot easier than to live a healthy lifestyle of discipline and self-control, for discipline and self-control require strong willpower, and not everybody has it. Their favorite excuse is to bring out some famous chain-smokers and reckless adventurers who live a long life as their role models. They ignore the fact that they are rare exceptions. They also ignore the grim prospects of bad health that affect themselves and their families until they are seriously ill, which usually is too late for them to make any changes. I can relate to their sentiments because I know so many people who don't drink, smoke, nor eat junk foods, and they also live a very healthy lifestyle by exercising regularly. Yet still, they acquire those awful illnesses such as cancer, diabetes, heart, and other rare diseases, which cut their lives short. I am also aware of the fact that most of the foods we eat are either loaded with harmful chemicals or genetically modified, and they are not good for us. Just go to the internet, you will find endless articles telling us "Not to eat this and not to eat that," and if we believe in them, we can't eat anything at all and we'll be starved to death, because they are everyday items, such as breads, fruits and vegetables, things we must eat in order to survive. Of course, many of these articles use scare tactics to scare us into buying their products. But, the facts they present are also quite true. And that's scary! If we keep on destroying our environment, modifying our food for bigger profits, and doing nothing to reverse the trend, we'll see the end of the world, wiped out by our own hands with our advanced technologies and smart inventions as weapons. The sad thing is we, as an individual, can do nothing about it. To save our world, we need the cooperation of every single one of us, and I don't believe it's possible.

So, I believe in fate and believe that when it is time for us to go, we must go. But, I believe in statistics more. There is no denial, according to numerous reliable studies and researches, that smokers are more likely than non-smokers to have lung diseases, that heavy drinkers have liver diseases, that junk food eaters and exercise haters develop diabetes and obesity, and that risk-takers suffer more injuries and incur more accidents. Therefore, be realistic, and do all those things that are under your control and live a clean, healthy life, and trust your life in the hands of fate. Although fate might still work against you, you can be assured that the chances of attaining good health, longevity, and a happy life are much better.